NOURISHING BALANCE

A Journey to Wellness

Alex Owen

ISBN-9798398249989

Cover design by: Art Painter

Library of Congress Control Number: 2018675309

Printed in the United States of America rights reserved.

DEDICATION

This Book is dedicated to my daddy Mr Emmanuel Owen who help me to become what I am today

Contents

Chapter 1: The Awakening

Sarah's realization that she current eating habits are negatively impacting her well-being. She decides to educate herself about nutrition, seeking out reliable sources of information and consulting professionals. As Sarah woke up to yet another morning of fatigue and lethargy, she couldn't help but feel a growing sense of frustration. Days seemed to blend together, filled with moments of low energy and a lack of vitality. She yearned for a change, a way to break free from the grips of exhaustion that had become all too familiar.

One afternoon, as Sarah sat on her couch, mindlessly snacking on a bag of chips, a sudden wave of realization washed over her. She recognized the direct link between her eating habits and how she felt daily. It was as if a light bulb had switched on in her mind, illuminating the path to a healthier, more vibrant life.

Determined to uncover the truth about nutrition and its impact on well-being, Sarah set out on a quest for knowledge. She realized that relying on convenience foods, processed snacks, and sugary treats had taken a toll on her body, leaving her feeling depleted and unwell. It was time to take charge and make a change.

Sarah's first step on this transformative journey was to educate herself. She delved into books, scientific studies, and reputable online resources, seeking out reliable information about nutrition. She understood the importance of separating fact from fiction, avoiding the traps of fad diets and quick-fix solutions. Sarah craved a deeper understanding of the impact food had on her body, mind, and overall health.

Recognizing the complexity of the subject, Sarah decided

to seek guidance from professionals in the field of nutrition. She scheduled appointments with registered dietitians and nutritionists, eager to gain personalized insights and expert advice. These professionals helped her navigate the vast sea of dietary information, offering practical tips and evidence-based recommendations tailored to her specific needs.

Sarah's understanding of nutrition grew with each conversation and resource she explored. She discovered the essential role of macronutrients, such as carbohydrates, proteins, and fats, in providing energy and supporting bodily functions. She learned about the importance of micronutrients, like vitamins and minerals, for overall health and well-being. Sarah began to grasp the significance of balanced meals, incorporating a variety of whole foods into her diet.

Sarah's awakening to the impact of her eating habits was not merely a fleeting moment of insight. It sparked a fire within her to transform her relationship with food and reclaim her vitality. She realized that her journey would require patience, commitment, and a genuine desire for change. As Sarah closed the chapter on her old eating habits, she embarked on a new chapter of self-discovery and empowerment. The awakening had set her on a path of nourishment, where she would learn to fuel her body with wholesome, nutrient-dense foods. The decision to educate herself and seek guidance from professionals marked the beginning of a remarkable transformation—one that would lead her to a life filled with energy, vitality, and a renewed sense of well-being.

In the subsequent chapters of "Nourishing Balance: A Journey to Wellness," join Sarah as she dives deeper into the fundamental principles of nutrition, unveils common myths and misconceptions, and builds a foundation of knowledge that will empower her on her quest for a balanced and nourished life.

Chapter 2:

understanding the Basics

Sarah delves into the fundamental principles of nutrition, learning about macronutrients, micronutrients, and their importance for the body. She becomes familiar with food groups, portion control, and the significance of balanced meals. Armed with a newfound determination and a thirst for knowledge, Sarah delved into the world of nutrition, eager to understand the fundamental building blocks of a healthy diet. She realized that to achieve nourishing balance, she needed a solid grasp of the basics.

Her journey into understanding the basics began with an exploration of macronutrients—the essential components of food that provide energy and perform vital functions in the body. Sarah learned that carbohydrates were the primary source of energy, supplying fuel for physical and mental activities. She discovered that proteins played a crucial role in building and repairing tissues, while also supporting the immune system and various metabolic processes. And she understood that fats were not to be feared but rather embraced in moderation, as they aided in nutrient absorption, protected vital organs, and provided a concentrated source of energy.

In addition to macronutrients, Sarah delved into the realm of micronutrients—vitamins and minerals that were required in smaller quantities but were equally vital for maintaining optimal health. She learned about the various vitamins, such as vitamin C for immune function and vitamin D for bone health, as well as minerals like iron for oxygen transport and calcium for strong bones and teeth.

As Sarah continued her exploration, she encountered the concept of food groups, which served as a practical framework for creating well-balanced meals. She familiarized herself with the different food groups, including fruits, vegetables, whole grains, lean proteins, and healthy fats. Understanding the role of each group allowed her to design meals that incorporated a variety of nutrients, flavors, and textures. Portion control also emerged as a key component in Sarah's understanding of the basics. She realized that it wasn't just about the types of food she ate, but also the quantity. By learning about appropriate portion sizes, she could ensure she was consuming adequate nutrients while maintaining a healthy weight.

Sarah grasped the significance of balanced meals, which comprised a combination of macronutrients and micronutrients from various food groups. She discovered that a balanced plate consisted of colorful vegetables, lean proteins, whole grains, and a small portion of healthy fats. By incorporating a variety of foods into her meals, she could ensure she was obtaining the essential nutrients her body needed to thrive.

Armed with this newfound knowledge, Sarah felt

empowered to make informed choices about her diet. No longer would she view food as mere sustenance, but rather as a means to nourish and fuel her body. She understood that achieving a nourishing balance was not about strict diets or deprivation, but rather about creating a sustainable and enjoyable lifestyle centered on wholesome and nourishing foods.

In the subsequent chapters of "Nourishing Balance: A Journey to Wellness," Sarah's understanding of the basics would continue to evolve. She would learn to decipher nutrition labels, explore the concept of mindful eating, and uncover the truth about processed foods. Join Sarah as she applies her growing knowledge to build a foundation of healthy eating habits and further advance on her path to wellness.

Chapter 3:

Unveiling the Myths

Sarah encounters common nutrition myths and misconceptions that hinder her progress. She uncovers the truth behind fad diets, food trends, and conflicting information, distinguishing fact from fiction.

As Sarah delved deeper into her journey of nutrition and wellness, she encountered a barrage of conflicting information, fad diets, and sensationalized food trends that promised quick fixes and miraculous transformations. It became evident to her that navigating the world of nutrition required a discerning eye and a commitment to uncovering the truth.

In Chapter 3, "Unveiling the Myths," Sarah embarked on a quest to separate fact from fiction, aiming to dispel the misleading beliefs that had held her back and hindered her progress thus far. She confronted one of the most pervasive myths in the world of nutrition: the idea that restrictive diets were the ultimate solution to achieving health and weight loss. Sarah discovered that fad diets often provided short-term results at best, leading to a cycle of weight loss and regain. She realized that restrictive eating patterns were not sustainable in the long run and could even harm her overall well-being. Instead, she sought a balanced and flexible approach that would support her health and happiness for the long haul.

Sarah also encountered the misconception that certain foods should be entirely avoided or demonized. She learned that labeling foods as "good" or "bad" oversimplified the complex nature of nutrition. Rather than focusing on restriction, Sarah discovered the importance of moderation and mindful indulgence. By embracing a balanced perspective, she freed herself from the guilt and anxiety associated with certain foods and fostered a healthier relationship with eating.

Another myth Sarah confronted was the belief that one-size-fits-all diets were universally applicable. She realized that individual bodies had unique needs and that nutritional requirements varied based on factors such as age, activity level, and personal health conditions. Sarah understood the importance of personalized nutrition and the value of tailoring her dietary choices to meet her specific needs and preferences.

Throughout her exploration, Sarah encountered

conflicting information that left her feeling overwhelmed and uncertain. She recognized the importance of critically evaluating sources and seeking evidence-based information from reputable experts. By developing her skills in discerning reliable sources of nutrition information, she gained the tools necessary to navigate the ever-changing landscape of dietary advice. With each myth debunked, Sarah's confidence grew, and she became more adept at distinguishing fact from fiction. Armed with knowledge and a critical mindset, she was no longer swayed by flashy marketing campaigns or sensationalized claims. She found solace in evidence-based research and the wisdom of trusted professionals, enabling her to make informed choices that aligned with her goals and values.

In Chapter 3 of "Nourishing Balance: A Journey to Wellness," Sarah's mission to unveil the myths allowed her to shed the shackles of misinformation and embrace a more authentic and empowering approach to nutrition. Join her as she continues to uncover the truth and forge a path towards sustainable and evidence-based wellness practices.

Chapter 4: Building a Healthy Plate

Sarah explores the concept of mindful eating, discovering how to create a well-balanced plate with whole foods, fruits, vegetables, lean proteins, and healthy fats. She experiments with new recipes, incorporating nutrient-dense ingredients into her meals. In her quest for nourishing balance, Sarah realized that building a healthy plate was an essential step towards achieving her wellness goals. Chapter 4, "Building a Healthy Plate," became a pivotal chapter in her journey as she embraced the concept of mindful eating and discovered the power of nutritious, whole foods.

Sarah learned that creating a well-balanced plate meant incorporating a variety of nutrient-dense ingredients. She recognized that whole foods—unprocessed or minimally processed foods—formed the foundation of a nourishing diet. These foods provided a rich array of vitamins, minerals, fiber, and other essential nutrients that supported her overall health and well-being.

Fruits and vegetables took center stage in Sarah's plate-building adventure. She discovered the importance of incorporating a colorful assortment of fruits and vegetables, as they provided a wide range of nutrients and antioxidants. From vibrant berries to leafy greens, Sarah learned to appreciate the diversity and flavor they brought to her meals. She experimented with different cooking methods and recipes, exploring new ways to make fruits and vegetables a delightful and integral part of her daily menu.

Lean proteins also played a vital role in Sarah's healthy plate. She understood that proteins were essential for building and repairing tissues, supporting muscle health, and promoting satiety. Sarah explored various sources of lean proteins, such as poultry, fish, legumes, and tofu, and incorporated them into her meals. She learned the value of portion control and the importance of balancing proteins with other food groups to create a harmonious plate.

Recognizing the significance of healthy fats, Sarah sought to include them in her meals as well. She discovered that fats were not to be feared but embraced in moderation. Healthy fats, such as avocados, nuts, seeds, and olive oil, offered a host of benefits, including supporting brain health, absorbing fat-soluble vitamins, and providing a feeling of satisfaction. Sarah learned to incorporate these fats into her dishes mindfully, balancing their inclusion with the overall composition of her plate. Sarah's exploration of building a healthy plate extended beyond just individual ingredients. She also discovered the importance of portion sizes and mindful eating practices. Sarah learned to listen to her body's hunger and fullness cues, savoring each bite and eating with intention. This newfound awareness allowed her to enjoy her meals more fully and prevented overeating or mindless consumption.

Throughout her journey, Sarah embraced her creativity in the kitchen. She experimented with new recipes and cooking techniques, discovering delicious ways to incorporate nutrient-dense ingredients into her meals. She found joy in preparing meals that were both nourishing and flavorful, realizing that healthy eating didn't have to be bland or monotonous.

Chapter 4 of "Nourishing Balance: A Journey to Wellness" became a turning point for Sarah as she learned to build plates that not only provided nourishment but also delighted her senses. Join her as she continues to refine her skills in plate-building, exploring new flavors, and finding fulfillment in the art of creating nutritious and delicious meals.

Chapter 5:
Understanding Individual Needs

Sarah learns about personalized nutrition, considering factors such as age, activity level, and specific dietary requirements. She discovers how to tailor her nutrition plan to meet her unique needs and preferences. As Sarah delved deeper into her journey of nutrition and wellness, she came to understand that one-size-fits-all approaches to nutrition were inadequate. Chapter 5, "Understanding Individual Needs," became a crucial chapter in her quest for nourishing balance as she explored the concept of personalized nutrition.

Sarah discovered that numerous factors influenced an individual's nutritional needs. Age, activity level, metabolism, genetics, and specific dietary requirements all played a role in determining the ideal balance of nutrients for optimal health and well-being. With this knowledge, she recognized the importance of tailoring her nutrition plan to meet her unique needs and preferences.

To begin her exploration of personalized nutrition, Sarah assessed her age and life stage. She understood that nutritional requirements evolved throughout life, from childhood to adulthood and beyond. Sarah learned how to adapt her diet to support her changing needs, whether it be for growth and development, maintaining energy levels, or supporting healthy aging.

Activity level emerged as another significant factor in understanding her individual needs. Sarah recognized that physical activity influenced her energy expenditure and nutrient requirements. She learned to fuel her body appropriately, considering the duration, intensity, and type of exercise she engaged in. Sarah discovered the importance of consuming adequate carbohydrates for energy, sufficient protein for muscle repair, and appropriate hydration to support her active lifestyle.

Additionally, Sarah acknowledged that specific dietary requirements, such as food allergies, intolerances, or medical conditions, played a crucial role in shaping her nutrition plan. She sought guidance from healthcare professionals, such as registered dietitians or doctors, who helped her navigate these unique considerations. With their expertise, Sarah developed strategies to accommodate her specific dietary needs while still enjoying a varied and balanced diet. Sarah embraced the power of self-awareness, recognizing that personal preferences and cultural influences impacted her relationship with food. She learned to honor her individual tastes, incorporating foods that she genuinely enjoyed into her meals. By finding a balance between her preferences and nutritional requirements, she fostered a sustainable and enjoyable approach to eating.

In Chapter 5 of "Nourishing Balance: A Journey to Wellness," Sarah's understanding of individual needs expanded beyond the surface level. She considered a holistic view of her well-being, recognizing that her mental and emotional health also influenced her nutrition choices. Sarah explored mindful eating practices, stress management techniques, and self-care strategies, all of which contributed to her overall wellness.

Join Sarah as she continues her exploration of personalized nutrition, understanding that she is unique and deserving of a nutrition plan that supports her individual needs and empowers her to thrive on her path to nourishing balance.

Chapter 7: The Mind-Body Connection

Sarah explores the connection between nutrition and mental well-being. She discovers the impact of certain foods on mood, stress levels, and cognitive function, and adopts practices like meditation and self-care to support her overall wellness. In her quest for nourishing balance, Sarah uncovered an essential aspect of well-being: the profound connection between nutrition and mental health. Chapter 7, "The Mind-Body Connection," became a transformative chapter in her journey as she delved into the interplay between what she ate and how she felt.

Sarah recognized that her food choices could significantly impact her mood, stress levels, and cognitive function. She discovered that certain nutrients played a vital role in supporting brain health and balancing neurotransmitters responsible for regulating emotions. Sarah learned that consuming foods rich in omega-3 fatty acids, such as fatty fish, walnuts, and flaxseeds, could potentially alleviate symptoms of depression and anxiety. She also explored the benefits of antioxidant-rich foods, like berries, leafy greens, and dark chocolate, which could protect against oxidative stress and promote mental well-being.

Moreover, Sarah understood the importance of managing stress and its impact on her overall health. She discovered that chronic stress could disrupt digestion, hinder nutrient absorption, and contribute to inflammation in the body. Sarah explored various stress management techniques, such as meditation, deep breathing exercises, and mindfulness practices. These practices allowed her to cultivate a greater sense of calm and awareness, promoting both mental and physical well-being.

In her exploration of the mind-body connection, Sarah also recognized the role of self-care in maintaining optimal health. She understood that nourishing her body extended beyond just nutrition. Sarah learned the importance of taking time for herself, engaging in activities that brought joy and relaxation. Whether it was practicing yoga, enjoying nature walks, or indulging in a soothing bath, Sarah discovered that self-care rituals were essential for restoring balance and promoting a positive mindset.

Through Chapter 7 of "Nourishing Balance: A Journey to Wellness," Sarah continued to deepen her understanding of the intricate relationship between nutrition and mental well-being. She embraced the power of food as a tool for supporting her mental health, while also integrating practices like meditation and self-care to nurture her mind and body.

Join Sarah as she explores the mind-body connection, discovering the transformative effects of nourishing her body with wholesome foods, managing stress effectively, and cultivating self-care practices to support her overall wellness. Together, let us unlock the powerful synergy between nutrition and mental health on the path to nourishing balance.

Chapter 8: Sustainable Habits for Life

Sarah embraces a long-term approach to nutrition, focusing on sustainable habits rather than short-lived diets. She establishes routines for meal planning, grocery shopping, and food preparation, ensuring she can maintain her newfound healthy lifestyle.

As Sarah's journey toward nourishing balance progressed, she came to a significant realization: true wellness was not achieved through short-lived diets or quick fixes but through sustainable habits for life. Chapter 8, "Sustainable Habits for Life," became a pivotal chapter in her quest as she shifted her focus from temporary changes to lasting lifestyle transformations.

Sarah understood that sustainable habits were the foundation of maintaining her newfound healthy lifestyle. She recognized that consistency and moderation were key to achieving long-term success. Instead of strict rules or rigid guidelines, Sarah sought to create flexible routines that seamlessly integrated nourishing habits into her everyday life.

Meal planning became one of Sarah's cornerstones for sustainability. She discovered the importance of prepping her meals in advance, ensuring she had nutritious options readily available. Sarah dedicated time each week to plan her meals, taking into consideration her schedule, dietary preferences, and nutritional needs. By doing so, she minimized the likelihood of resorting to unhealthy choices due to time constraints or lack of options. Meal planning empowered Sarah to make mindful decisions about her food, fostering a sense of control and satisfaction.

Accompanying meal planning, Sarah developed the habit of strategic grocery shopping. She learned the importance of creating a shopping list based on her planned meals, focusing on whole foods and nutrient-dense ingredients. Sarah became mindful of reading labels, prioritizing fresh produce, lean proteins, and whole grains. By practicing conscious grocery shopping, she cultivated a supportive environment at home, filled with nourishing options that aligned with her wellness goals.

In addition to meal planning and grocery shopping,

Sarah recognized the value of food preparation. She discovered that spending time in the kitchen, experimenting with new recipes and preparing her meals, offered numerous benefits. Not only did she have control over the ingredients she used, but she also found joy and fulfillment in the process of creating nourishing dishes. Sarah honed her cooking skills, exploring various cooking methods and flavors, ensuring that healthy eating remained exciting and enjoyable.

Throughout Chapter 8 of "Nourishing Balance: A Journey to Wellness," Sarah focused on establishing sustainable habits that would support her for a lifetime. She understood that true transformation required consistency, patience, and a willingness to adapt to life's changes. Sarah embraced the idea that sustainable habits were not restrictive or burdensome but rather empowering and liberating.

Join Sarah as she discovers the joy of sustainable habits, adopting routines for meal planning, grocery shopping, and food preparation that fit her lifestyle. Together, let us cultivate sustainable practices that nourish our bodies and ensure a lifelong commitment to wellness.

Chapter 9: Sharing the Journey

Sarah becomes passionate about sharing her knowledge and experiences with others. She starts a blog or support group, inspiring and guiding others on their own nutrition journeys.

As Sarah's own transformation unfolded, a newfound passion ignited within her — the desire to share her knowledge, experiences, and insights with others. In Chapter 9, "Sharing the Journey," Sarah embarks on a mission to inspire and guide individuals on their win nutrition journeys.

Recognizing the power of community and the value of support, Sarah sought to create a platform where she could connect with like-minded individuals. She decided to start a blog or support group, a space where she could share her story, offer practical tips, and foster a sense of camaraderie among those seeking to improve their well-being.

Through her blog, Sarah chronicled her personal experiences, from the challenges she faced to the triumphs she celebrated. She shared her knowledge of nutrition, offering evidence-based information in a relatable and accessible manner. Sarah provided guidance on meal planning, recipe ideas, and strategies for overcoming common obstacles. Her blog became a source of inspiration, encouragement, and motivation for others embarking on their own wellness journeys.

Additionally, Sarah established a support group where individuals could come together to share their struggles, successes, and insights. This community provided a safe and judgment-free space for members to seek guidance, ask questions, and celebrate milestones. Sarah facilitated discussions, offered expert advice, and encouraged the group to support and uplift one another.

Through her blog and support group, Sarah discovered the power of connection and the incredible impact of inspiring others. She witnessed individuals finding solace in shared experiences, gaining knowledge and confidence to make positive changes in their lives. Sarah's journey of nourishing balance became a catalyst for transformation in the lives of those she reached.

In Chapter 9 of "Nourishing Balance: A Journey to Wellness," Sarah's passion for sharing the journey reached its pinnacle. She recognized that her own growth and progress were enhanced through the act of empowering others. Sarah became a beacon of inspiration, guiding individuals toward a nourishing and balanced life.

Join Sarah as she opens her heart and shares her wisdom, creating a supportive community where individuals can find encouragement, guidance, and the tools to embark on their nutrition journeys. Together, let us inspire and uplift one another as we strive for nourishing balance in our lives.

Chapter 10:

Flourishing in Wellness

Sarah's dedication pays off as she experiences increased energy, improved health markers, and a newfound zest for life. He reflects on her transformation, expressing gratitude for the positive impact nutrition has had on her overall well-being. In the final chapter of "Nourishing Balance: A Journey to Wellness," aptly titled "Flourishing in Wellness," Sarah emerges as a shining example of the transformative power of nutrition. Her unwavering dedication and commitment have led her to experience a life filled with vitality, improved health, and a renewed sense of purpose.

Through her journey, Sarah has witnessed the positive impact of her nutrition choices on her overall well-being. She wakes up each day with increased energy, ready to embrace the opportunities and challenges that come her way. Sarah's fatigue has been replaced by a vibrant zest for life, allowing her to fully engage in her passions and pursue her dreams with the subjective experiences, Sarah's commitment to nourishing balance has yielded tangible results. She undergoes regular health check-ups and celebrates the improvements in her health markers. Whether it's lower cholesterol levels, stabilized blood sugar, or a healthy weight, Sarah's body has responded positively to her mindful nutrition choices. She recognizes the role that nourishing her body plays in preventing chronic diseases and enhancing her overall quality of life.

In Chapter 10, Sarah takes a moment to reflect on her incredible transformation. She expresses gratitude for the positive impact that nutrition has had on her physical, mental, and emotional well-being. Sarah acknowledges the challenges she faced, the lessons she learned, and the growth she experienced throughout her journey. She is proud of the choices she has made and the person she has become.

Moreover, Sarah recognizes that her journey doesn't end with her transformation. She is inspired to continue advocating for the importance of nutrition and well-being. Sarah becomes an ambassador for nourishing balance, sharing her story, knowledge, and insights with others. She continues to uplift and support individuals on their wellness journeys, empowering them to unlock their full potential and flourish in their own lives.

In the concluding chapter of "Nourishing Balance: A Journey to Wellness," Sarah stands as a testament to the transformative power of nutrition. Her story serves as a beacon of hope and inspiration for others seeking to create positive change in their lives. Join Sarah as she reflects on her journey, expresses gratitude for her transformation, and embraces a life of flourishing wellness.

Together, let us celebrate the power of nourishing balance and the incredible potential we all have to create vibrant, healthy, and fulfilling lives.

Chapter 11: Embracing Nourishing Balance

In the final chapter of "Nourishing Balance: A Journey to Wellness," we reach the culmination of Sarah's transformative odyssey. This conclusive chapter, "Embracing Nourishing Balance," encapsulates the essence of her journey, offering a profound reflection on the power of nutrition and its profound impact on overall well-being. As Sarah stands at the precipice of her journey, she gazes upon the path she has traversed with a mixture of gratitude and awe. The challenges she faced and the lessons she learned have shaped her into a stronger, more resilient individual. Sarah's once-fleeting dreams of vitality, vibrancy, and fulfilment have blossomed into a beautiful reality through the nurturing power of balance.

In this final chapter, Sarah delves deep into her personal growth and transformation. She reflects on the profound shifts in her mindset, the unwavering commitment she made to herself, and the invaluable knowledge she acquired along the way. Sarah celebrates the triumphs, both big and small, and acknowledges the setbacks as essential stepping stones on her path to wellness.

But it is not only Sarah who has benefited from her journey. Through her vulnerability and determination, she has become an inspiration to those around her. Friends, family, and even strangers have witnessed the remarkable changes in Sarah's life and have been moved to embark on their transformative quests. Sarah's story has become a catalyst for positive change, lighting the way for others who seek to find their nourishing balance.

In this conclusive chapter, Sarah expresses profound gratitude for the power of nutrition and its influence on her overall well-being. She acknowledges the intricate dance between mind, body, and soul, understanding that true wellness is a holistic experience. Sarah celebrates the nourishment she has provided not only to her body but also to her spirit, cultivating self-care practices, and embracing a newfound sense of self-love.

As we bid farewell to Sarah's transformative journey, we are reminded of the universal truth that nourishing balance is not a destination but a lifelong endeavor. It is a continual dance of making mindful choices, adapting to new circumstances, and embracing the ebb and flow of life. Sarah's story serves as a reminder that every individual has the power to embark on their journey, nourish their bodies, and embrace balance in their unique way

The closing of "Nourishing Balance: A Journey to Wellness" is not an end but a new beginning. It is an invitation for readers to embark on their odyssey of self-discovery, armed with the knowledge, inspiration, and guidance they have found within these pages. Sarah's story will forever be etched in their hearts as a beacon of hope, reminding them of the incredible potential that lies within.

So, dear reader, as you turn the final page, know that the power to embrace nourishing balance resides within you. Let Sarah's journey be the catalyst for your transformation. Together, let us embark on a lifelong quest to nourish our bodies, minds, and souls, and to create a life filled with vitality, purpose, and joy. Embrace the nourishing balance that awaits you and step into a future of limitless possibilities.